WAD THE F*CK

WAD THE F*CK

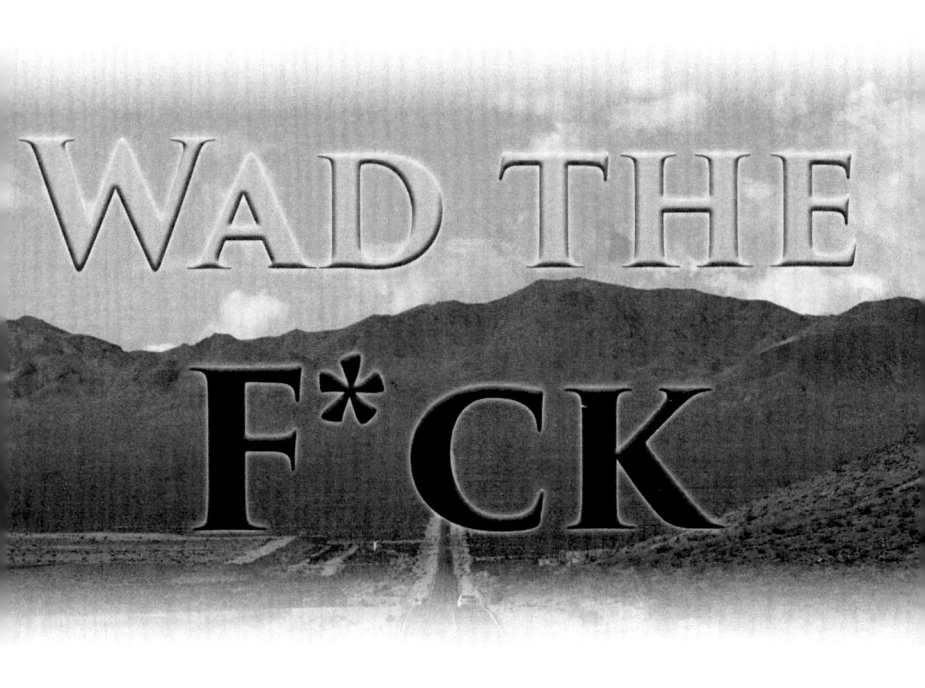

Whiplash Shelley

WAD THE F*CK

Copyright © Shelley Wrona, 2023

All rights reserved. No part of this publication may be reproduced, stored in a retrieval system, or transmitted in any form or by any means, electronic, mechanical, photocopying, recording, or otherwise, without written permission of the author and publisher.

Published by Shelley Wrona, Edmonton, Canada

ISBN:
    Paperback   978-1-77835-201-0

Publication assistance and digital printing in Canada by

PAGEMASTER
PUBLISHING
PageMaster.ca

Happy Definition

- favored by luck or fortune
- enjoying or characterized by well-being and contentment
- expressing, reflecting, or suggestive of happiness
- having or marked by an atmosphere of good fellowship
- enthusiastic about something to the point of obsession

Merriam-Webster
https://www.merriam-webster.com › dictionary › happy

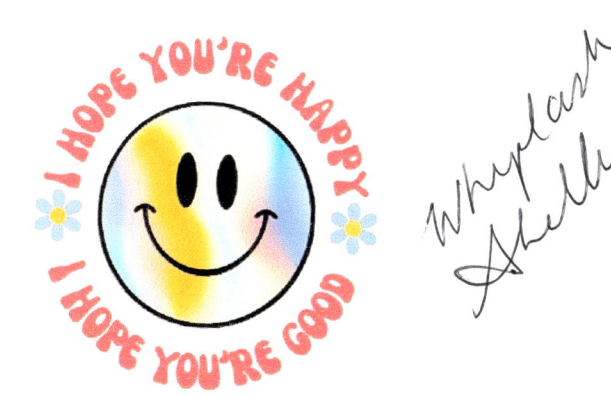

Contents

Starting Line: August 2017 5

An Accident Occurred...human error 6

Whiplash
Definition: 9

Cue music... 13

The Physio Package...needles included 19

Referral to a physiatrist....hmmm interesting title 45

Door #4 55

Just say no to drugs... 61

Analyze this...psychology...
how does that make you feel? 65

We've booked you an IME Bitch... 73

Botox...not just for celebrities 77

I Cancelled My Car Insurance Policy...
and House Insurance Policy 81

Friend...such a simple word
 for one of the great necessities of life 83

Finish Line: 85

Starting Line: August 2017

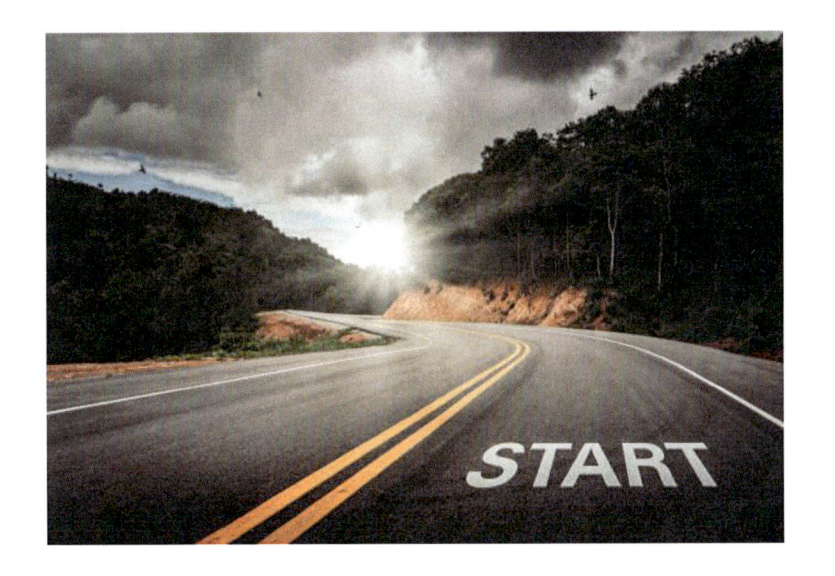

An Accident Occurred...human error

*

I had just finished work and was driving home. The season was the summer and the weather was full sun! Traffic was light, my tunes were on spot and I was thinking about all the things I needed to get done for my daughter's wedding. Less than a month away and I had lots to do still; Plus, I was still going to lose 40 lbs LMAO!

I was close to home and waiting at a yield sign. There were two cars to go by me and then it was my turn. My turn didn't quite happen though. Instead, a guy hits my car from behind. I was stopped, not moving or going to move until the cars passed. Why did he take his foot off the brake pedal and switch to the gas pedal? I wasn't even inching up to get ready to go. The hit wasn't at a high speed, but enough to move my car ahead from where I was stopped.

The hit from behind occurred and my head first went forward then back. No time to react or brace myself. I have often thought "If I wasn't so relaxed it may not have gone the way it has." But nobody knows how each person does with an injury. I loudly said, "WTF!" All I thought, was, "I don't need this right now." I looked ahead to see a car pulling over who was a witness to this accident. I got out of my car and listened to the guy, who hit me, yell that I should have gone! Question, WHAT? After yelling he turned to look at his car, you know, to make sure it was okay. Having the witness came in real handy...he corrected the guy in road rules/safety. We did the exchange of paperwork, took pictures, and then left to go home. No "sorry" or "hope you're okay" was exchanged from the guy who hit me. This guy's yelling at me did not sit well. He was clearly in the wrong, but if yelling made him feel good, so be it; you were still in the wrong, my friend.

When I got home, I noticed that the back of my head kept stinging. The stinging is what I felt very first after the hit. I called my car insurance company to ask what the procedure is after a minor accident like mine. On this initial call, I was told my car insurance rates would go up. I was quite sure this lady didn't really seem to know what she was talking about. Best I take care of my head, then get back to them. In the meantime, I texted my man friend who was an RCMP. He told me what to do and most importantly why to do it. I then went to the walk-in Medi-centre in Spruce Grove that early evening. I saw a physician who did an examination (no gown) and said I had mild whiplash and it may get worse over the next three days.

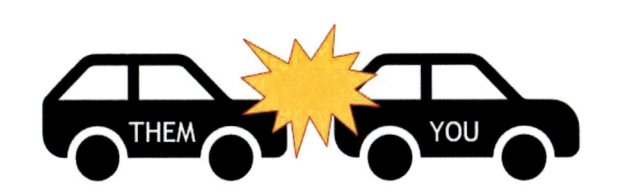

I was also advised to report this accident to our local RCMP department, which I did. I also made the appointment to have my car fixed. The damage was only $1000 which I had fixed so the transmission could be looked at. The car was good and only received a new shiny bumper.

Here's my journey about a whiplash injury. This journey had me explore my emotional well- being. A small accident at a low speed, but shook my happy world into a constant state of pain for over 5 years. These are my words and my feelings. My name has been changed to protect me- actually that's a big fat lie. I changed my name to 'Whiplash Shelley' at some point into Year 2 because it sounded really cool and gave me more power over the injury in a silly, but meaningful way. I hope you enjoy the read.

Whiplash Definition:

*

What is whiplash? It is a short-worded definition, which I find a little amusing, because of the collection of symptoms that can occur following damage to the neck.

Whiplash is the term used for the **force** that causes the injury and not for the injury itself. The injury is **neck pain** and other symptoms it can cause.

It is a common type of neck injury and happens when the neck jolts backward or forward, sharply and suddenly. Whiplash due to a motor vehicle collision can strain muscles or damage soft tissues in your neck.

I have it and despise it. My neck pain has been caused by whiplash; it's the worst kind of overachiever. And it wasn't just centralized to my neck. It radiated throughout my upper body and affected my shoulders and arms, as well as my head; for me, it produced headaches of which I had many. Don't forget some TMJD; pain in the jaw. Neck/shoulder/jaw pain interferes with your day-to-day activities. Your sleep is affected and spending time with friends and family becomes a chore that you choose to just ignore sometimes. I mixed pain, lack of sleep and distance from friends, and found myself in a gloomy/depressing place at times.

There is no doubt in my mind that I have dispelled any myths and misconceptions I had about this common, yet invisible injury. Whiplash is real and the pain is real.

They classify Whiplash-Associated Disorders (WAD) by the severity of signs and symptoms:

- Grade 0: no complaints or physical signs.
- Grade 1: indicates neck complaints but no physical signs.
- Grade 2: indicates neck complaints and musculoskeletal signs.
- Grade 3: neck complaints and neurological signs.
- Grade 4: neck complaints and fracture/dislocation:

I had a Grade 2 WAD with the following collection of symptoms that occurred as a result of the automobile accident: injury to my jaw (TMJD), frequent headaches, dizziness, insomnia, fatigue, tinnitus, loss of focus, some depression, irritability, injury to intervertebral joints, cervical muscles, nerve roots, neck stiffness, injuries to the muscles and ligaments (myofascial injuries), sensations such as burning/stinging in head, and shoulder pain.

I would say Year 1 and 2 were the absolute worst for the above symptoms and all the treatments I explored. I almost had a full-time job driving from one appointment to another. It was crazy and I was crazy miserable for a lot of this time. Now, passing the 5th year of this journey, it isn't hard to recollect or go back in time and think about the pain. And, if my math is correct, 5 years and a bit is over 60 months, but I remember it vividly- my pain. I remember being so tired all the time and feeling like a complete failure. I remember the pain that started in my neck and shoulder after about 5-10 minutes of driving and dreading to change lanes, fearful I might hit someone because it hurt to shoulder check. I remember the last time I mowed the lawn.

Cue music...

✱

Before we start, let me talk about something I absolutely love and helped me throughout this journey. Music. Love it to death.

Music is a powerful catalyst. Music can transform the emotions and feelings of people with vocal or instrumental sounds. It can lessen stress, pain, distraction and bring positivity and calmness into our day.

"I hope the place has good music." That's what I always said if I was going to any kind of appointment that had office background music. There's nothing like sitting in the waiting room with crappy music or worse, no music. It can make or break the atmosphere. It's the worst for me.

I love to listen to music during work, outside in the yard, driving anywhere and falling asleep to some nice relaxation instrumental sounds.

So happens my father loved music. Probably where I got my love of it from, or least I like to think that. I grew up listening to a lot of his genres of music, but was never really fond of the country genre he played quite often. It wasn't until I had my own records and listening to the radio, I figured out I really, really, really still didn't like country music.

Whenever my father came out for a visit, he would always "bline" to my CDs/cassettes or records. He would spend time to look at all of them and then pick some to play. One Christmas tradition was my dad buying me and each of my siblings a record he knew each of us would like. This was the only time there was no sibling rivalry, pretty much. It's only in the last few years that I really got how much my dad really loved his music and how it attaches to my memories of him now. If I put on one of his records now, I know which songs off the album are my favourite. So, I think I did like some of his music! My iTunes collection includes some of his favourites.

My listening to music has increased quite a bit these last 5 years as my music library as well. I got to enjoy more music due to lots of time on the highway going to appointments and in appointments/waiting areas. It's probably what kept me sane. With the music on, mood got good and what would be a bad day looked brighter. There are days, very few mind you, but yes some days I don't listen to any music. My genres are most everything, but heavy on alternative rock. Maybe a wee bit of country now as I am giving it one more shot! Damn you, country music!!

Parkland Physiotherapy has music playing all the time. I love it- just a good feel to the start of your day in my opinion. I've downloaded lots of new songs from my visits there and on one particular night I heard a song that really caught my attention. Blue October is the band. "I Hope You're Happy" is the song. Immediate download and immediate obsession with this song and the band. This song has been played almost every day for five years and sometimes it will go on repeat! After I downloaded the song, I began to read about the band

Blue October. I liked what I read. A story of lead singer, Justin Furstenfeld, getting back up after time with an addiction of drugs and alcohol. I've always liked seeing or hearing of people that have had addiction and are in recovery. Like how it happened, maybe why it happened and how their journey was to get to recovery. Success stories- that's what they are. I became totally obsessed with the band, but not enough to drive people crazy with it.

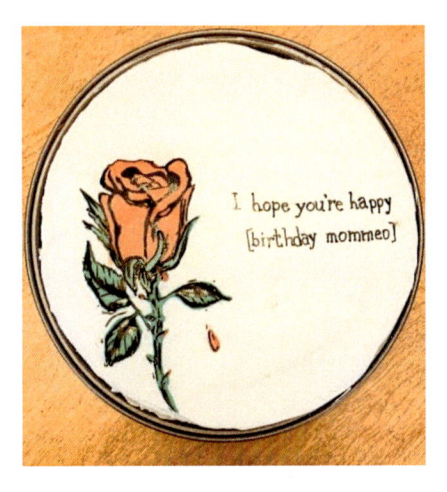

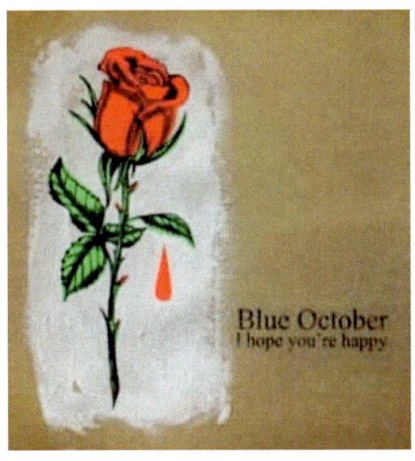

I was lucky enough to go see them in concert in June 2019. My friend and I went to Anaheim House of Blues. I had a meet and greet package. It included sound check, open conversation with the band, picture with the band, then...the signing of my poster lmao!!! I also had the lead singer sign my arm.

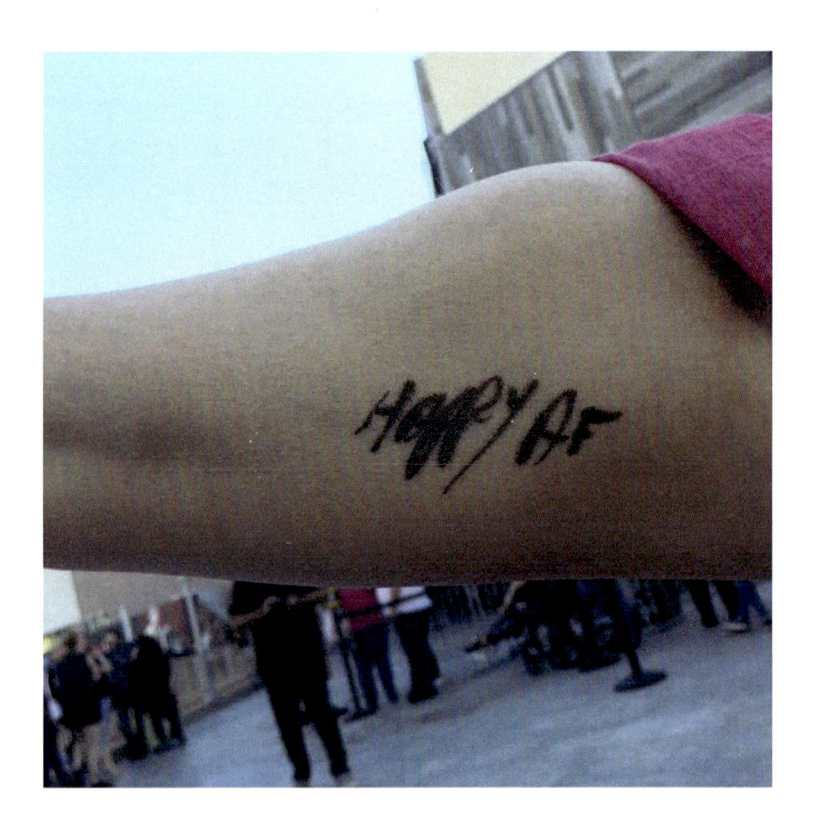

The concert was fabulous!!! More fabulous than when I saw the Bay City Rollers in the early 70's and the drummer, Derik, gave me his scarf!

I did have to sit part way through the concert as I was getting sore, but that was just fine, I still saw the concert on the big screen sitting in a comfy couch at the House of Blues. We both had just a fantastic time-some more great memories.

They have released a few more albums out since my obsession began and all I can say is their music just gets better and better.

I was going to change careers and uproot my life to go be a roadie with the band, but since COVID, I don't think it's going to happen, but more concerts and meeting the band will though!

The Physio Package...needles included

*

The physician who told me it was mild whiplash and that it may get worse the next 3 days or so, was quite right, the stinging in my head was constant and the start of a sore neck and headaches began on Day 3 or 4. My friend said, "You should go to physiotherapy" and to, "call sooner than later" something about you only have a 10-day window to get treatment started. Well holy crap it's Day 7, best I call. So, who to call...the only one I really knew of without googling was Parkland Rehabilitation Physiotherapy, attached to the Tri Leisure Centre in Spruce Grove. You can't miss it. It's a big place that has been there since I can remember. I called and was given an appointment within the allotted time frame for insurance purposes.

Before I continue, let me give kudos to the front desk staff, each and every one of them. During all of my treatment appointments at Parkland Rehabilitation Physiotherapy I have had the absolute pleasure of never having to hear some answering machine telling me to Press 1, 2, 3, etc. to make/change/cancel an appointment and listen to the recording carefully because "their" options have recently changed.

Seriously, I think I would have lost my shit if I was having to call to book an extra appointment and sit on hold pressing buttons with a bad headache. If you were to walk in, you are greeted at the main reception desk, with a smile or an eye roll (you know who you are)! The process of checking in and out is seamless, efficient and, if needed, they go the extra step to accommodate your needs if they can.

The consultation went well. The atmosphere there was inviting/good vibe and music was good (that was a big deciding factor). I was given a mild whiplash diagnosis then made appointments and bada-boom, bada-bing, lets' fix 'er up shall we!!

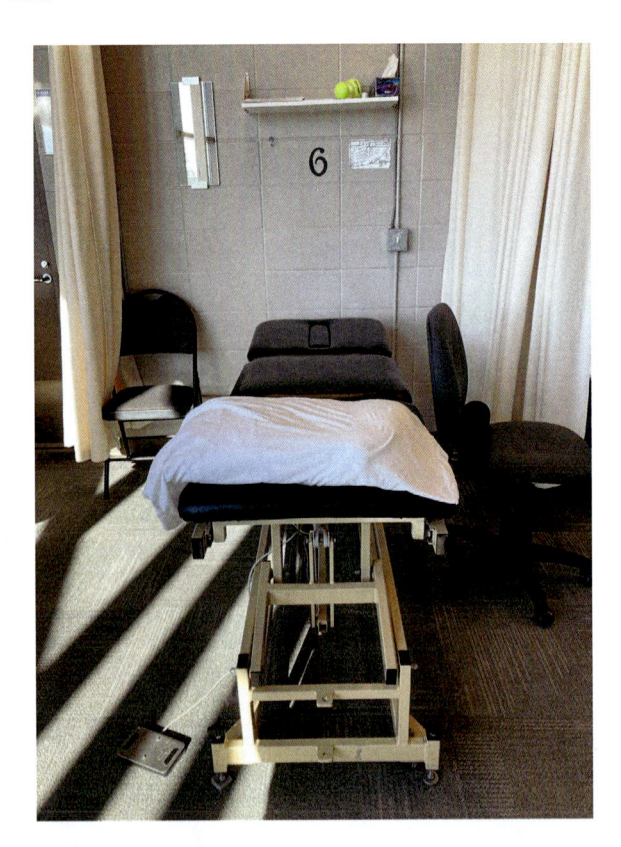

At the consultation appointment I did need to mention I had my daughter's wedding in 4 weeks and a holiday to Disneyland booked in 6 weeks. I didn't plan on changing my trip to Disney, that's for sure. It was much needed. The wedding came quick, as my extra time was now fitting in some physiotherapy appointments around work. The wedding was beautiful and I somewhat coped with my headaches with lots of Advil. Nobody could tell I had a headache for 4 days- wickedly good stuff, that Advil. Now for the second conundrum, how am I going to the happiest place on earth and not do any rides-am I going to be better? Well, it ended up I wasn't better. It hurt a lot even doing the one or two rides I managed to do on this trip in September 2017. A set back, but I was totally disappointed and sad. I've been to Disneyland 7 times since the accident. Prior to the accident I had been about 15 times so I am a well-seasoned guest at the parks and most of the rides!! Throughout this journey I did learn to turn some of the negative experiences (doing the rides) into a positive. My thoughts focused that the next time was going to be better! I did "next times" a lot and each next time was going to be my "comeback" and I was going to enrich my mind in a place I absolutely love. I did have to learn over these last few years to make my trips enjoyable with or without some of my favourite rides. I still believe there will come a time I will be 100% and it'll be one big celebration in Disney. That celebration may include the cutest grandson who absolutely loves MM! And just to be crystal clear about my travel during this journey, it was never easy for me. I had, and continue, (when needed) to use other means to help me out during the travel. It always included pain relief with medication, but also, I improvised with things that wouldn't aggravate the neck. You get good at knowing ahead of time what is going to do what to the neck or shoulders-right down to the type of purse you would carry. But I did have to ask for help along the way. I didn't really like doing that. During my Disneyland trips I became acquainted with their first aid offices. One in California Adventure Land (it's on the left-hand side when you first walk in) and in Disneyland, The Golden Horseshoe (across from the steam boat) is where I use a couch to lay down and the crushed velvet curtains as my pillow! I am happy to report that I have not laid down in the last few trips now. I rest up in the form of sleep if I can and before I go to the park that day, I use a hot pack- I never miss packing a hot pack. And the most important task is to have physiotherapy as close to my leaving date as I can. This is the Disneyland package, good.

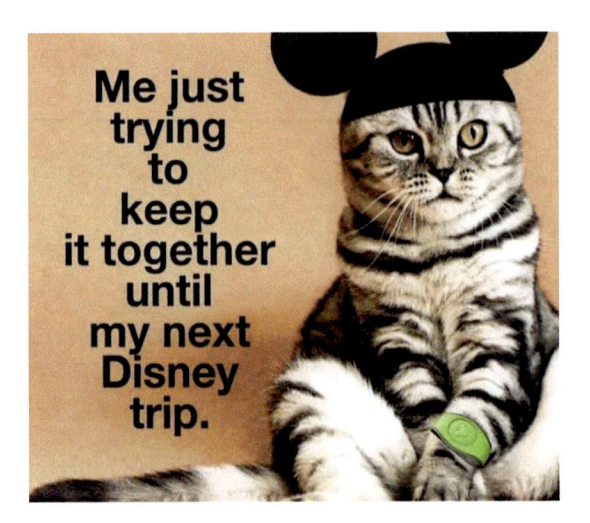

> Mar 10, 2013
>
> Hi. You have reached Shelley and Jamie. We aren't able to come to the phone right now because we are in DISNEYLAND!!!!!!! Please leave a message and we will call you back when we grow up!!

Initially when given a Grade 2 that included neck complaints I also experienced a host of other symptoms during this journey, as I listed under the whiplash definition. When these other symptoms would appear, I would report them to the physiotherapist and other medical professionals and would eventually need to see so we could deal with them. Never, ever, did I think I would have more than a soft tissue injury with this accident. I thought 3 to 4 months max. for physiotherapy treatment. I think I missed the memo with the time frame of recovery.

So, let's go to physio shall we! Initially I would go early, like 6:30 am or 7:00 am appointments, then I could go to work right after. Now I am waking up earlier, packing clothes for work then flying to work after the appointment to keep somewhat of a normal schedule. It really was far from normal. I was so sleep deprived. I don't remember many days I woke up for work or an appointment being happy. All I knew was I had to go, I had to get ready and that made me not so happy, actually miserable is what it made me. I despised morning routine now, getting ready through pain. Many times, I would be getting up after a couple hours of sleep because the nerve pain had unleashed

23

during the night. I remember many early mornings getting to the physio place and parking, then dreading which I thought was an incredibly long walk to the front doors. I wanted to stick my thumb out and hitch hike to the front doors or have someone come get me in a wheelchair. Those front doors were less than a half a block from where I parked my car, actually maybe 100-200 feet. I just knew I was incredibly tired. But I got to any appointment and put on the face and got treated, at least that's what I did most of the time for many months. I probably thought I would blubber cry if I really said how I was.

I kept thinking that this was just a dumb schedule to keep for treatment if I wanted to get better. It hurt so bad driving to work after any physiotherapy appointments or any other procedure appointments, all I felt was I had just reversed the treatment and some or any positive effect it gave me. My two biggest instigators of the pain were driving and looking right. All my neck pain was on the right side. Any time I engaged my trapezius muscles, I felt the pain. Anytime I went shopping looking up or to the right at the shelves in the stores, gave me pain. I started shopping less and less. When talking to people they had to be in front of me. I remember my level of irritability was 10/10 when I had to ask a person twice to talk to me standing in front of me.

On the second ask, my neck was already in pain. Most days driving to or from work I wanted to pull over and lay down in the back seat of my car- just to take the engagement of my head and shoulders to a resting stage where the pain lessened. By the time I got home from work I was beyond miserable, I went straight to the bed and laid down until the pain would go away enough to get up and do a little bit around the house. I had to stop doing a lot of home stuff, the overwhelming need to lay down always won. I wasn't being lazy or sloth-like. And, I always thought, "this injury is going to clear up soon, I can catch up on stuff later." I had lots of days after coming home from work, I would watch the clock so I could just go to sleep early and have more time to heal. Lots of times the clock only made it to 6:30pm and I said, "f*ck it" and went to sleep, or tried to. I was usually up until 2 or 3am most nights.

I wasn't watching too much TV or on my phone when I was up late. I usually just laid in bed and was left with lots of thoughts running through my mind about things I needed to do. Sometimes I would get up and wonder around the house and try to stretch the muscles, maybe make a tea or a couple of voodoo dolls of people I was starting to not like much. I don't know how I got up for work most days, but I probably thought I would be so exhausted the next day and by the time night time came around, the sleep would come easier. It did not. The frustration of this interrupted sleep cycle was on another level for me. I have always been used to sleeping very well. I loved sleeping and getting up early feeling refreshed! I could fall asleep on a bed of rocks, that's how good I was at sleeping!

I kept this said 'dumb appointment schedule' for about a year. I finally asked my family doctor for a note. Don't ask me why I carried that schedule so long, I think I felt a lot of guilt missing work. And pain has a way of making its' own time clock; time went by fast in the first year. The note allowed me to stay home after any physiotherapy appointment or other medical appointments. I usually worked from home for a few hours after an appointment, but it was dependent on how I felt. Guilt usually dictated how much work I did too. And the guilt grew and grew and I worked more and more on my day away from the office.

I still book my appointments a little on the early side. One reason is to have little absence from work and the other is the feeling I look forward to after a successful session. It's like flying in on my broom and driving home in a Porsche!

After 6 months into Physio, actually way before that, I will say I looked high and low for quick fixes to lessen the pain. I was desperate and consumed with getting rid of the pain. None of the devices/OTC (over the counter) meds I bought ever worked. Big time disappointment every time and my frustration only heightened. I always believed relief was right around the corner or on some late night I would see an infomercial with a miracle fix. I missed very few scheduled physiotherapy appointments. I did what was asked or suggested and tried to keep up with my overall wellness at the same time. This was not easy at all. The amount of pain was so overwhelming at times. I would have three good days and then wham; Mr. Pain came knocking. Who let you in and why? What is going on? How do I outsmart this creature of pain?

I always use to gauge my recovery process without the pain on certain things I did or the time in hours or days until the pain came back. When that came, oh was I ever happy, but, oh when the pain came back was I ever not happy. My mind was totally consumed with the feeling of no pain and how long before the pain came back. I think I wasted that time. Was it worry or overthinking? Probably a bit of both and it was time I plain wasted. Pain doesn't text or send you an email. It just shows up, just like that.

To me that was the kicker, I didn't understand it. I need to read up on this and how muscles recover from an injury. I need to be in the know now and get a grip on this. I don't want it to be gripping me like this. Initially I had a diagnosis of WAD II. When another diagnosis came my way after a consultation with the physiatrist, I wasn't too happy. Chronic myofascial pain syndrome.

This is a medical term used to describe muscle pain and referred pain. My referred pain kept landing in the same spots, neck and shoulder. The tight muscles in knots, known as trigger points become inflamed and painful. It hurts a lot. I can't imagine doing this type of pain long term. I used to ask or as some call it, bitch, to the therapists, "are we there yet? Like, when is this done? How much longer!" They must get that question a lot. There are many factors in the healing process and we cannot do much to control the physiological healing time of our body tissue. There are different rates of healing and a quick fix was not reality. Once I realized this, I stopped asking and gave that energy somewhere else. I gave the energy to understand better the pain cycle and what I looked like in it. My goal was to get out of this cycle, the healthy way.

I would see the same therapist at each visit, Cam. If he wasn't available then I saw Tayo or Ben. All very experienced in their profession and have obviously kept up their certification in humor! Cam has the knowledge, positivity with good listening and interpersonal skills. He never wavered from the treatment and was engaged with other treatments I would have. It really did prove the best pathway for healing and wellness.

So, what happens at your appointments? Well, I'm glad you asked! I can tell you I never put a gown on, just a nice stretchy shirt. No gown, good. You know what else is good at Parkland Physiotherapy, the physiotherapy aides. Your appointments are not only greeted with smiling faces at the front desk, but you get another lovely person to check you in and escort you to the section/bed for appointment. They will fetch you a hot pack and sometimes you may have some time for a brief shits and giggles session. Keeping the good vibe!

So, yes, each appointment starts with a heat pack around my neck/shoulders. I LOVED this heat and loved it more after any IMS sessions (dry needling).Those heat packs were toasty hot and I started to need the immediate heat affect so no white towel became the normal. Just a heat pack with a liner. Get that heat in.

The first 12 weeks was 2-3 times a week and then it worked its' way down to once a week per the protocol I assume. I assure you I was there more than what the protocol road map looked like. There were quite a few times I would go extra when a bad headache reared or a really bad episode of pain would not go away. I remember having twice the anger when I had to get another appointment. I had to switch stuff around with work and that was not easy. I had a lot of responsibility with my work and I never wanted to disappoint anybody.

After the first 12-16 weeks of the average recovery time for a mild whiplash came and went, the weeks started to stretch into months and more, years. Having passed the 5-year mark I can honestly say I know where the time went. It went where it should have, getting better and leaving the pain behind. The recovery point for me isn't everyone else's. I am definitely different in terms of what and how I feel every day prior to the accident and the best thing is that I am happy with it now. *I got "me" to my better and got happy with it now.* I see how the process works with pain and how you become, but when the pain lessens slowly, but surely, maybe not a 100%, you become somewhat a better version of your old self because inside you are so *thankful*. Not throwing in the "towel" was key for me and giving it time.

Home stretches/exercises were also key in the recovery process. I did them. I did not do them when I was in pain. Remember…my pain and my experience with this pain. And have a good cervical pillow, no bad reviews from mine, love it. Even if you do not have neck pain, I would highly recommend a good cervical pillow. Keeps your neck and spine in alignment, restful sleep and improves posture. The cost is a little bit more than your average pillow, but a good investment.

Here are some tools/equipment and tricks of physio. Actually, there are no tricks at all. Physiotherapy is to restore, maintain, improve your mobility and function and a mind and body of well-being.

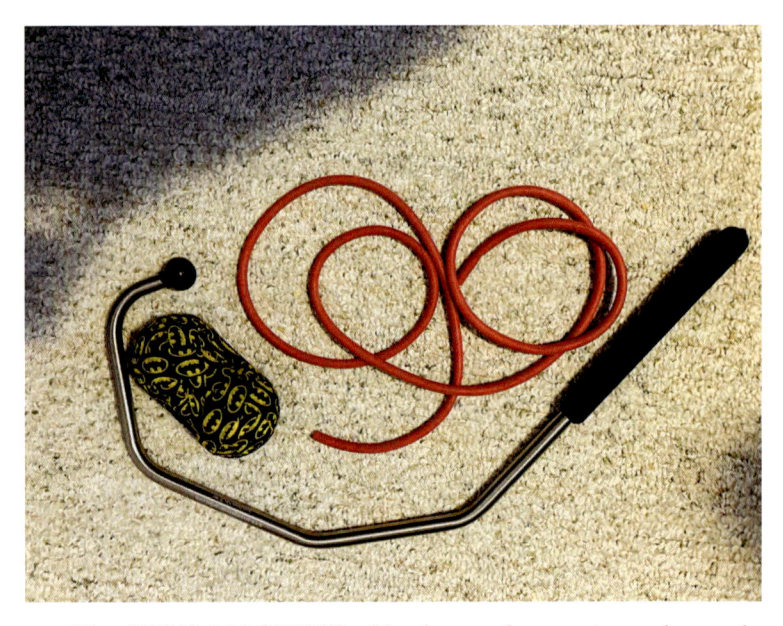

The **TENS MACHINE:** Used to reduce pain and muscle spasms. It's a small, battery-operated device that has leads connected to sticky pads called electrodes. There is the use of a mild electrical current and is a good method of pain relief I found. You would place the sticky pads where needed and turn the machine on to desired pulse/current. I had that on the shoulders and head area. I really, really liked it a lot. It was like waves of water pulsating over the muscles pleading with them to just f*cken relax!! Having muscle spasms or really tight muscles in your head is no picnic, I had them so bad sometimes it would wake me out of a sleep. I would need to get up, but I couldn't get out of a sleeping position unless I slithered on my stomach off the bed and slowly had my head relax so I could lift it. Most times I had to reach for some Advil and chase it with Sangria from Trader Joes. The head muscles were horrible, but my shoulder muscles clearly won the award for best, tight body muscle. I felt like a cow's ass looks: two huge muscles on either side of my neck. They were solid as a rock and full of pain. I was told your shoulder muscles should have the feel of a raw steak. I had a long way to go!

There was also **MASSAGE**. Everyone knows what massage is: the act of pressing, rubbing and manipulating your skin, muscles, tendons and ligaments. It can range from light to deep pressure. I hated massage from the beginning up until the start of Year 4 or 5. Until then it made me so nauseated. I don't know what the reasoning was behind the nausea, but as things progressed into a better state overall the nausea certainly subsided. When I did feel I was ready to onboard with some massage treatments I was given the best referral. I made an appointment to see Miss Jessica. An experienced lady in this field for sure. Tuned into my pain and really ready to incorporate the best path. I have been really liking this and have seen improvement since I started. I go twice a month for a regime of deep tissue massacre (I mean massage) some cupping technique (no flames) and more deep tissue massage. My curse meter was high in the beginning and has really tapered off now. I think it's really how I have gauged my pain- who needs rating scales! Actually, I do use rating scales at physio. I like them so I take that back, we should keep using rating scales out there! Miss Jessica also uses lots of oils too and CBD oil is included. Still no gown! I must say that I am getting good at refusing to wear a gown- in the politest way, of course.

I would highly recommend Miss Jessica. She loves and appreciates the feedback which always proves effective when addressing any injury. You can and should be your own health advocate and make decisions, do the reading and anything else you see need, but you really need to be onboard with dedicated, understanding healthcare professionals.

There was also a **TUNING FORK** (traditionally used by doctors to test for hearing) that came into the mix which was effective for my headaches. Who knew! To achieve this treatment modality, the physiotherapist brought the fork to a vibration state and placed the stem on the body part affected, my head. This experience was very relaxing. The ache in my head agreed.

The **TRACTION MACHINE** has become a fixture in most physiotherapy clinics. This form of traction gently pulls the head and stretches your muscles. It operates off a head halter and pulley system. First, you get on bed, put head in the head halter where it holds your head still and correctly positioned. Then turn the machine on and let it stretch you slowly. There is also a bed buzzer device you can hold on to, similar to a comfort blanket to a 2-year-old, if you needed to turn the machine off. Yes, I held it close to me. The first time I was shown how to stop the machine with the bed buzzer stopper, it fell apart. HILARIOUS!! Fast thinking prevailed and out came the electrician tape. That stuff fixes anything!! I wasn't a big fan of the traction machine, but, because traction is also thought to provide muscle relaxation by minimizing your muscle guarding and ultimately reduce muscle pain, I did participate when up to it. If there was a positive in the stretch machine, growing 2 inches taller was it! Kidding, I probably grew in places I didn't need.

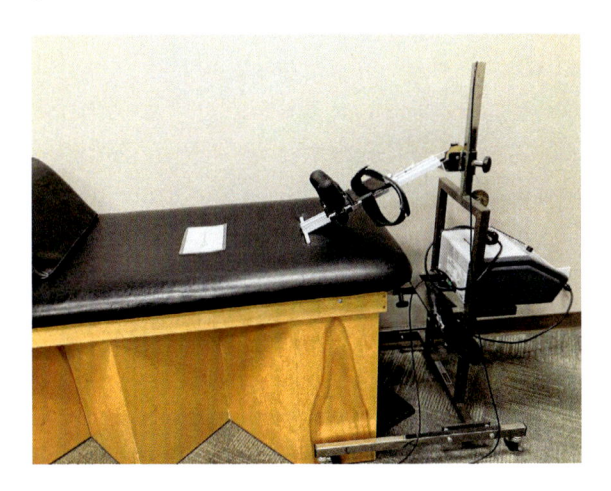

The **NECK HAMMOCK** was a newly developed device I found on the internet. This device was developed by a physiotherapist and looks and does exactly what it's called.

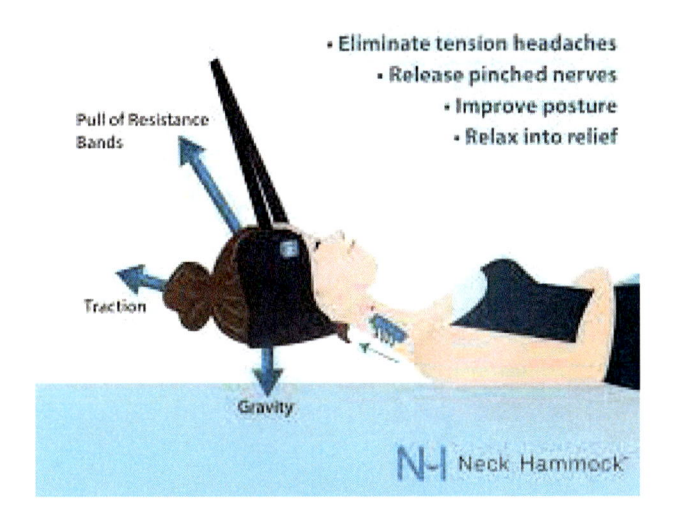

The neck hammock uses cervical traction to provide fast neck pain relief, and a faster recovery from neck injuries and is suppose to feel good when using.

I had Cam test drive this device and he gave his approval to use at home. I really failed this at all different time points I tried. I never felt comfortable when having my head hang in it. My focus was on getting the comfortable feeling it was to provide despite having issues that had not fully healed enough to get near the comfortable feeling. After many months of using or trying to use the neck hammock, I let the dust settle on the hammock, literally. I abandoned this completely and would re-visit when I was ready. I have re-started the neck hammock very slowly and am feeling better with the after effects of it. Should be a good staple to incorporate into the daily stretching regime.

Please, don't get me wrong. Each appointment wasn't like walking through a field of daisies. I had so many days I felt I was tangled in rose thorn vines with two horns coming out of my head. Some days not all the treatments worked and I would have to not use this or that for a time and then re-visit it later. There were lots and lots of days I wanted to cut my head off. I felt very strongly about this. To me it was the only solution, get rid of the problem. I've had the problem long enough. I don't want a long-term relationship with chronic pain. It's horrible. And no, obviously I didn't cut my head off but I was so miserable at times though even I didn't like me or things I was saying or thinking. The coping was agonizing. I tried hard to shift my really bad moods. Some days I just didn't give enough of a shit to shift shit anywhere, but at people I came in contact with. I did feel a sense of out of control when I would lip someone off or mimic their voice/talking because I was so spent with this whole thing. Just leave me be is how I felt. There were also the constant conversations with the insurance company.

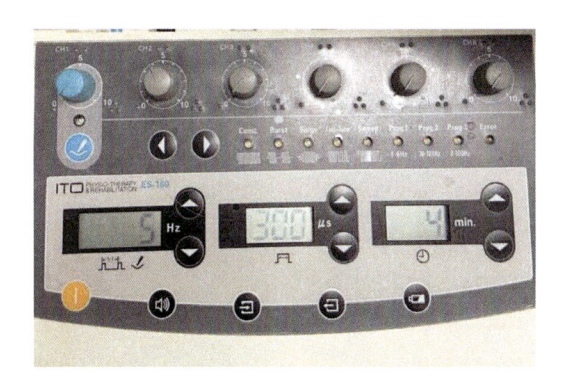

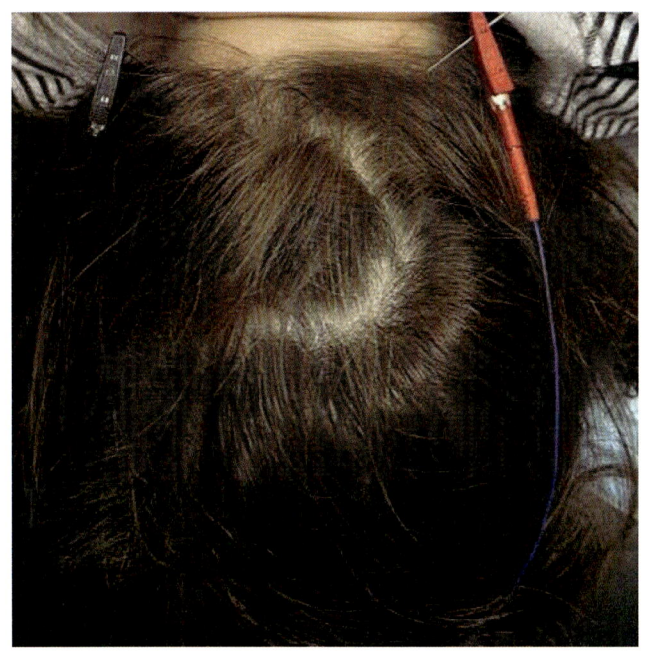

After weeks and now months of listening to this insurance agent guide me on when I should be healed and that it was my fault I wasn't healed already because I wasn't listening to the physiotherapist, I decided to not engage with her shit anymore. I should have done it sooner. The sound of her voice sent me over the edge some days, no, all days I spoke with her. Like nails on a chalkboard. By not engaging with insurance agent but still adhering to their rules etc. I was much happier and whatever happened would happen. I had no control over the insurance company and their ethics and morals.

Of course, over time, the coping became more and more manageable when I could gauge a significant shift in the pain. This part I just loved. It took time to get to a shift in pain and as long as I was going in this direction, I would keep walking the walk.

The needles in the base of head and machine are not IMS or dry needling, but it is called a **Electroacupuncture Unit ES-160**. In electroacupuncture this machine is attached to a pair of needles and a small electric current is passed through them. It wasn't the most comfortable feeling, but it did work on my tight muscles in this spot.

This next section I saved for last.

When I first heard of **IMS** or dry needling, I was like, "what? Needles? Sounds painful," and, "are you insane? What's the point?" I texted an RN and said, "they want to use needles, what do I say or do?" to which the RN replied, "I love needles!" That was the end of that text. I did a little googling on dry needling. In the physiotherapy world, it's a procedure used often. Yes, there is a lot of literature out there that reflects dry needling in a negative light and yes there are a lot of skeptics that pish-posh dry needling, but a 100% I say "don't knock it until you try it". And you know you would try a lot of different treatments when you suffer from pain and need relief of the immediate kind. Dry needling is not the same as acupuncture.

This became the mainstay of my treatment sessions.

My name is Whiplash Shelley and I love dry needling, but hate the pain. I have been dry needling since October 2017. No Airmiles or Optimum points collected, it's better than that... pain free muscles/trigger points.

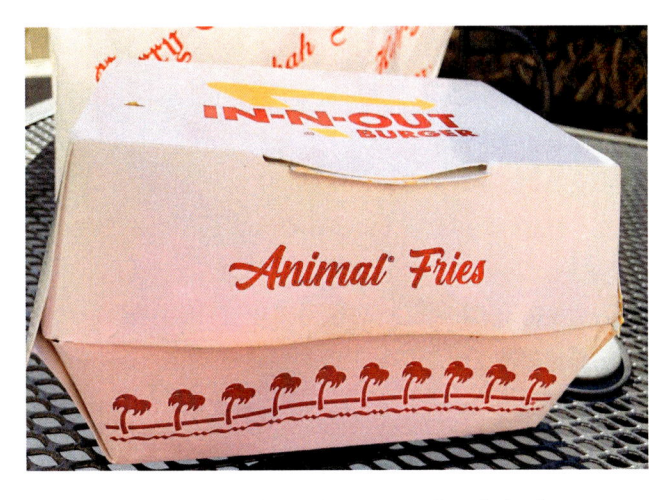

*Nothing to do with needles or pain but, I also love In & Out burger and their Animal Fries!"

Trigger Point Dry Needling involves the insertion of acupuncture needles into taut (pulled tight) bands of muscle (or trigger points), in order to elicit (make happen) a local twitch response. The twitch response causes relaxation of the muscle and an increase of blood flow in the area. The result to the lengthening of the muscle and increase in circulation combine to stimulate the body's natural healing process, was brilliant to my way of thinking. They say the insertion of a needle into normal muscle tissue is virtually painless, but the insertion of a needle into a shortened, taut band will produce a grasping of the needle by the muscle, which can be a more intense sensation. The intense sensation is referred to as bloody intense pain. It hurts, a lot. I think my muscles were so bloody tight that the needle went in, the twitch response turned on and went right to HIGH! There was always if not often an immediate improvement in my mobility, however there were lots of times I had leftover achiness in the muscle that persisted for approximately 24 hours. My heat pad had a lot of use on these days. I just had to remember to not over exert and start painting or gardening to mess up something someone had just straightened out.

The following explanation of IMS (Intra Muscular Stimulation) is taken from different websites I would read and each of the physiotherapists I saw. I tried to interpret and form into most of my own words so that you could understand what it is and what I experienced.

If someone asked me to explain a session, I would say the following:

You take an experienced physiotherapist, some long-ass needle filaments and one patient with tight muscles. And it goes a little something like this: the needles are poked (tapped) in and twisted through a muscle knot to get a response twitch. It's like untying a knot. That twitch or jump of a muscle fibre is painful. Like holy shitballs of fire, painful. My first session exploded with some colourful words, as would all or most further sessions. The anticipation of the needle going in and causing a boat-load of pain made me nervous each and every time. The pain was just straight up painful, but it only lasted a short amount of time, like a few seconds, but long seconds. These treatments had immediate effect with me. This isn't my best analogy, but it is like using a brush on your tangled hair; it can hurt a lot, until you put the detangler in and the brush strokes through your hair effortlessly. That's what the needles did for me. After the IMS was done, I could feel the tightness in the muscles turn into a more relaxed state. The fatigue was always overwhelming for me after each appointment, but I stuck with it. No point dilly dallying- this was my instant relief from pain. My thoughts usually zeroed in on being one needle away from pain! My guide/pain meter for a successful treatment with IMS was usually later on in the day or the next day. I felt more relaxed, less tightness in the shoulders/back of head muscles and in my jaw. Yes, we did the jaw area and back of head. Wasn't that painful? Did you cry? Whiplash Shelley doesn't cry, but she can guarantee it was painful. Remember your chronic pain feeling is so focused on a result, relief. One of my best places to have IMS was to the side of the head, known as the temporalis something or rather, this muscle would or became tight when I had a doozy of a headache. I loved the feeling the IMS produced as I felt the needle do its' thang. It was like a wave of water going through my temple. I could have those all day long and never swear! There were so many sessions where I felt happy first then I would feel less pain, less frustration and less anger/irritability. The IMS sessions were very miracle like to me. And, well, I was in need of some miracles, the pain free kind. There was no getting around the fact that dry needling just worked for me, I just needed lots of it. The regular spots of the head were in the suboccipital area, along the neck and the trapezius area and of course the jaw.

Each physiotherapist, and there were three that worked on me, had a musician and/or song analogy of their IMS technique I gave them. Cam was like AC/DC Thunderstruck; Tayo was House of Pain Jump Around; Ben was Bruno Mars 24K Magic (smoother than a fresh jar of Skippy)

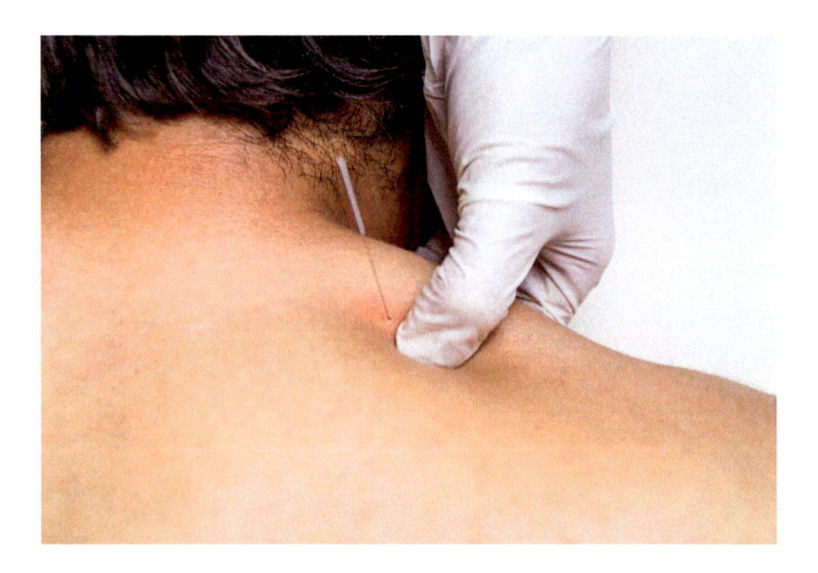

For my TMJD, which was diagnosed in December 2017, I was also referred to a dentist in the city. I definitely remember the consult being a painful one. My jaw, only on right hand side, was so full of pain and felt weak/tired/fatigued. I wished I could just scoop out the muscles in the area that was affected and be done with this pain. I went through the usual x-rays and some teeth moulds so they could make me a splint. The splint was a removable dental appliance that covered my lower teeth. The splint was intended to provide relief from pain and help relax and balance the jaw joints and muscles. I had many visits for re-alignments so the appliance was doing its' job. I was also having the dry needling of the jaw done consistently for added relief and with the intention of stopping long term pain. The dentist (such a lovely man who is so good at what he does) approved of the dry needling, very much. He was impressed and said, "whatever you are doing is working, keep it up." I would eventually stop wearing the appliance during the day and move on to the night mouth guard. This was to keep my jaw in the correct position and prevents grinding and clenching. I don't think I grind, but maybe I clench at night. The mouth guard was more to keep my jaw in the correct position and not have my back teeth hit each other which really did provide relief at night. Only thing was, I don't really like this appliance, a lot of the times I take it out during the night and look for it in the am. I find it hard to make this a habit.

During one physiotherapy appointment I remember I was having my jaw needled. All of a sudden, I felt an electrical jump go right through my eye. I absolutely lost my mind with pain. It felt like the needle went right through my eyeball. There was a burst of one bad, bad word (f*ck) I said 3 times, very loudly. I already have a loud voice so I am sure the next town over heard me. I was so close to the waiting room too. I felt horrible for this outburst. This is not good for their business. But, quick thinking and quick to his feet Cam went to the waiting room and anybody still left in their chairs, heard him tell them that everything is okay. From that day on I promised to cut out my cursing. It has lessened, not ceased. The believable excuse to myself is the way my brain and pain controls are wired; bad pain equals bad word. Then I feel better. And no, no kids were harmed when I was around. They know all the curses anyhow.

> Cursing raises our pain tolerance by about 50%.

These IMS treatments allowed me to do the stretching/exercises more effectively until things got tight and painful again. I had a long cycle of big pain and relief. Without the relief needling gave me, I don't know what state I would be in. Myofascial pain/trigger points are nasty. They feel like a burning ball of hot lava crossed with African killer bees under your skin. The inflammation and tightness of muscles that puts a person into pain overload sometimes, is overwhelming to say the least. It was horrible when I had out of control pain episode. I never knew when a wack of pain was coming my way. I never knew what I had done to trigger it, but some of these episodes reminded me of grey clouds dumping rain on my parade. And the thing is when that intense pain did stop, I felt a wee bit normal and relieved, mostly relief. I just wanted to get closer and closer to normal, just be normal.

When COVID-19 hit, everything closed for at least three months where I live and after that there were many starts and stops to opening again for business as a province. Besides the uncertainty of everything going on around us, I was at a little bit of a loss with things and not having needling handy. I am certain my muscles sort of relied on this service, I know I did. But people acted quick and soon enough the power of video calls were being used. A great tool, but unless you were a hairdresser 8 weeks into the pandemic, we were looking a little shaggy! I adapted to the video calls for physiotherapy as well as not driving to work. And maybe I will get ahead of the pain with a good break from driving too. I will say that the video calls were a good way to keep yourself in check/responsible for doing the work, I liked that.

I can end this chapter with these thoughts: Physiotherapy is such an important part in our healthcare system. This particular centre has carved out a business model that provides exceptional service with all their treatment modalities, except their hydrotherapy treatment. You couldn't pay me any amount of money to hop in a pool at this stage of my life, to have treatment of whatever kind. May as well hook me to some weights and let me go down.

My Google Published Review:

Small wreck and hurt my neck
Time for physio, off I go
Pick one close by, the one by the Tri-Leisure that is...Vibe is good.
Staff is cool. Music on spot.
Can't argue with hours but no candy bowl with sours
Physiotherapists know their stuff
But crap this is tough.
Go with the education provided, knowledge shared and advice given. They are humerus too, make no bones about that!
Fractures or bruises, bonks to the head,
post-op help or a massage to get back on track
Parkland Physio has your back

Referral to a physiatrist...hmmm interesting title

※

I am going to send you to see a physiatrist said my family doctor. I had never heard of a physiatrist, which in my line of work it seems I should have, I worked a bit with them. Maybe I didn't really have a good grasp on what they did. The biggest difference between physiatrists and physical therapists is the amount of education and training they receive. A physiatrist is a licensed medical doctor that has completed medical school and residency training in the specialty of physical medicine and rehabilitation. Both practices know the body's musculoskeletal system, however, a physiatrist's training allows for better knowledge about the structure and function of the body. Additionally, as licensed medical doctors, physiatrists have the authority to prescribe medication and perform surgical and nonsurgical therapies.

My first encounter with the physiatrist was in the spring of 2018. I had my initial consult with a third-year intern. That was the most colourful discussion and exam, as I was not expecting the exam to be as painful as it was. Felt bad for being as vocal as I was, but I honestly had no choice. There is a test they do to see if the nerves in your neck are crowded/irritated. It's called the Spurling test. The Spurling test is a medical maneuver used to assess nerve root pain (also known as radicular pain). The physician turns your head to the affected side while extending and applying downward pressure to the top of my head. I almost lost my mind with pain. I wanted to punch him right upside the head or put him in a headlock. This test makes the top 3 on my pain list. After this intensively painful visit, the physiatrist came in and established I have some neck issues. He goes on to talk about some options we could do. Go on, you have my attention.

First was some X-rays and a bone scan. Okay, I can do that. Not too invasive and no gown required, I don't think. I will call this Door #1. So off I go and have some x-rays of neck region, it did hurt because of the position they need you in to get a good "picture". The bone scan did not hurt but, the sneaky technician made me put on a gown, of which I did not like. Laying still was somewhat uncomfortable, but this was going to be a quick session and then they can read all the results and I'll know in a week or so. X-rays and bone scan came back unremarkable. This was good; I was good to go, knowing there was nothing sinister in these radiographs. Now, onto Door #2. The prize behind this door was some muscle numbing drugs. The physiatrist spoke to me about injecting a numbing agent such as Lidocaine or Marcaine into the area where my trigger points were. Let's describe trigger points again. They are sensitive areas of tight muscle fibers that can form in your muscles after an injury. A trigger point in a muscle can cause strain and pain throughout the muscle. When this pain persists and worsens, doctors call it myofascial pain syndrome. These drugs would be helpful to numb and relax the tight muscles. The first session of Marcaine was beyond marvellous. I was completely numb in all the areas I had pain. I'm like, "Mother, Mother May I take 8 steps forward, yes you may! Oh yes you may!!!" I drove home with the biggest smile! I'm so excited and I just can't hide it. Me and Marcaine had an instant connection. Love at first injection. This was my ticket I thought. My ticket to no pain and I was on the train- All aboard! When people win money, they imagine all the things they can buy now. I won a ticket that gave me pain-free stretching and other prescribed exercises. And I always knew each of these treatments outside of physiotherapy was not the "fix".

Each injection only lasted 8 hours or so and then wore off. It was a drawback, but 8 hours completely pain free took me back pre-accident where things were normal. And at this stage it's all I thought of. There were residual effects of the Marcaine/Lidocaine after the numbing wore off in that the muscles were not so tight so I could continue with some exercises. I also experienced headaches after the numbing wore off, but those were of the few kinds and wasn't the tension type. I continued with the injections and physiotherapy faithfully. Then after about 1 year of the injections every 2-3 weeks, the doctor decided to stop them as we weren't seeing as much benefit as he or I guess me, would have liked. I was really sad now. I was blaming myself for not doing better and trying to figure out where I went wrong. But muscle damage doesn't repair at the same time for every person. At the same time, I was having the trigger point injections the physiatrist had also referred me to have some shockwave therapy. I only ever had two sessions. Shockwave delivers targeted energy pulses and pressure waves directly on trigger points to help break up knots more precisely than can be done by a therapist's hands. Think of it like a wand/gun situated on your shoulders and continuous firing/pressure waves or like a jack hammer session. For me, it was horrific pain. I'm not sure if I had completed the shockwave therapy protocol if things would have been more effective with the trigger point injections, but I just couldn't go through this pain.

Imagine having a small cut on your finger. Just one cut and one finger. It is going to hurt a bit especially if something bumps the tiny cut or if you move your finger in just the right way. But the cut is nothing serious, just a small lived nuisance. Now, imagine your entire hand all your fingers have tiny cuts on them. These cuts are so numerous that they hurt, and hurt really bad. And since the cuts are so numerous, all your motions cause pain. This is the myofascial (covering of the muscle) pain syndrome. You have so many tiny muscle and fascial trigger points that your body's muscles are constantly in a painful state. Myofascial pain syndrome is a real bitch to treat I'm learning. The pain can be widespread that it can be difficult to know where to start.

So, now we had to talk about Door #3, and what was behind this door. Creak... (sound of door opening) You've won a Cortisone injection! Cortisone is common medicine injected for pain and inflammation and most commonly injected into joints. Well, it's not a new car or a trip, but I have some facet joints that could use some help in the pain department. I was explained the procedure. I did not like the sounds of this procedure. My biggest fear was being so close to the neck area where the pain is and using needles to get where it needs to be injected. After lots of thought and reading on it I agreed to do it and was referred to the pain control clinic that did this procedure.

It's at this curve in my road, I bid "adieu" to the physiatrist doctor. My treatment is switched to the pain control clinic who will be opening Doors 3, and possibly 4. I did have a hammer and box of nails on standby for Door #4 because I swore up and down, I would never open what was behind this door. No damn way. I was sad in a way to be leaving the care of this particular doctor, he was/is the real deal just being a genuine nice person/doctor.

My first appointment at the pain control clinic was to have a consultation with their pain doctor to see if I was eligible to have the cortisone injection. This physician performed a detailed history of my injury and a physical exam. Hmm, I may have some troubles with the gown scam I had going so far so I happily, but laughing my ass off, agreed to wear one when asked. She doesn't know I make voodoo dolls in the wee hours of the mornings when I am not sleeping. She agreed I would be a good candidate for the cortisone injection. But in order to have it I would have to have two nerve blocks first. The nerve blocks would report where exactly the pain is located. Why can't I just point to it? What's with all the high-level pain producing procedures on an already high pain output injury? I had not been preparing for the nerve block procedure. I had been watching quite a few videos on the cortisone injection procedure, but not the nerve blocks. When faced with this decision to have pain relief, but go through some more pain with the blocks, I was almost certain I would go ahead with it.

So here I go, nerve block one. You get prepped in the holding/recovery area. They get you to put a gown on (kill me now) and do your vitals etc. Then a lady comes and gets you and escorts you to the procedure room. She is the technician. She holds the fluoroscope (like a camera Xray) during the procedure to guide the physician to the precise area he needs to be with the needles. You get up on a normal table that has another mini mattress on it. It's half the width of the table. You lay face down. There is nothing to hold on to underneath the table and I know now this is going to be a challenge staying on the bloody table.

Doctor comes in. Doctor explains procedure. Shelley is told to hold still, absolutely no moving. Shelley does so. There is no freezing for this. Shelley may have forgotten this part of no freezing 3 seconds after being told. Shelley scared and Shelley initiates swearing. The needles are inserted and guided with the fluoroscope the technician is holding. You can feel every millimetre of the needle being guided and scrunched through muscle. Once at the spot, the confirmation is done with an injection of lidocaine. I am now feeling the lidocaine sting of a thousand bees and a boat load of pressure which subsided after 20 minutes or so. We have touchdown folks. This is the location of my pain. Now we know. Thankful it's over. *I did it.* I get up and wait a bit to make sure I don't have any complications then I walk out and drive home. I'm given a diary to record what I can do versus what I couldn't with the freezing in. Back on the lidocaine cloud! I was happy even it only lasted about 8 hrs. I had to wait a week or two before the next nerve block. Getting closer to the BIG injection!! See what I just did there. I turned negative into a positive!

Second nerve block went somewhat better. I think this doctor who was different from first block doctor, made the difference. Very attentive and talked to me before and during the procedure. The procedure was again a success. Pin pointed to same area. Walked out with gown on, still looking as ugly as can be, next time I need to gown up, I'll add a nice brooch.

I am now in countdown mode for the cortisone injection. And this couldn't have come at a better time. I had a work meeting in less than a week and didn't want to fly over 8 hours with the pain. My injection day came quick and I was so nervous. As I was walking to the procedure room, I had flash thoughts of how I got to this stage in treatment and wondering if this would be my last stupid gown I had to wear. I said my good mornings to the staff and picked my music. We have officially opened Door #3, let's go Bob. I laid down on my stomach on the procedure bed and gave a little prayer this time. In goes the needle crunching through muscles. The feeling of the needle, the guiding of it through you is such a gross feeling, I get the heebie-jeebies thinking about it still. There is some pressure with it too which was pretty much just another layer of uncomfortableness. The needles made it to the facet joints where relief was now seconds away. I was given the cortisone and felt it immediately. More pressure and a boat load of stinging pain. It wasn't immediate pain relief, and I remember that it took a day or two to kick in and cut the pain off. But I was able to exit the procedure room and inhale some more hope that this is it. And let's get that gown off; you look ridiculous, Whiplash!

I am in shape to attend a work meeting so off to London, England I go!! The first-class experience on the plane was pretty sweet. I never saw any royalty, but all the rave was goat cheese and goat milk ice cream and I had the chance to try A LOT of goat milk ice cream from the nearby market and goat cheese omelettes at the hotel. That may have been the highlight of that business meeting! Just kidding, the meeting was good, but truth be told, I actually found it hard to focus on this trip. I think I felt overwhelmed with the injection so close to leaving and maybe a little bit of worrying if something were to go wrong with possible side effect of the cortisone injection days prior. I was also thinking if I would be the nearing the end of all these appointments, all the driving I had to do, just all the stuff that kept going on whether I liked it or not, or whether I had control or no control of situations. What was going to change now? My four days at the meeting were not too bad in the physical manner, but I thought I would be numb like lidocaine gave me all those other times. It did not. But this is still a huge relief.

Well, it was a good run. We need to fast forward 5 weeks and I start to have pain. Pretty sure I know this pain from before. How can this be? It was supposed to last me up to 9 months. Now what. Now what the hell am I going to do? I'm devastated. I can't handle the shit. I did everything right and this procedure failed me.

I grabbed the phone a few weeks later and made an appointment with the physiatrist to get the referral, one referral I didn't want. He said the radio frequency nerve ablation is the last option now. This is Door #4. This is where I wanted to cry, scream, throw punches and kick walls. I felt I had no control, no choice or say in the matter. Feeling like that was one thing, but knowing was another, I knew I had choice and say, but I really saw it differently in that pain won this match and I would be opening one more door.

So off I go, back to the pain control centre to see pain doctor again. I had been watching video after video of procedure. I had a few questions and was almost mentally prepared. Then wham, pain doctor says you need two more nerve blocks. COME ON! Have you had a nerve block? How about I give you two blocks. One with the right hand and second with the left hand. I'm not going through them again. Please don't make me. She made me. We bartered and I only had to do one nerve block and I was approved for RFA.

Chronic pain is relentless agony.

Door #4

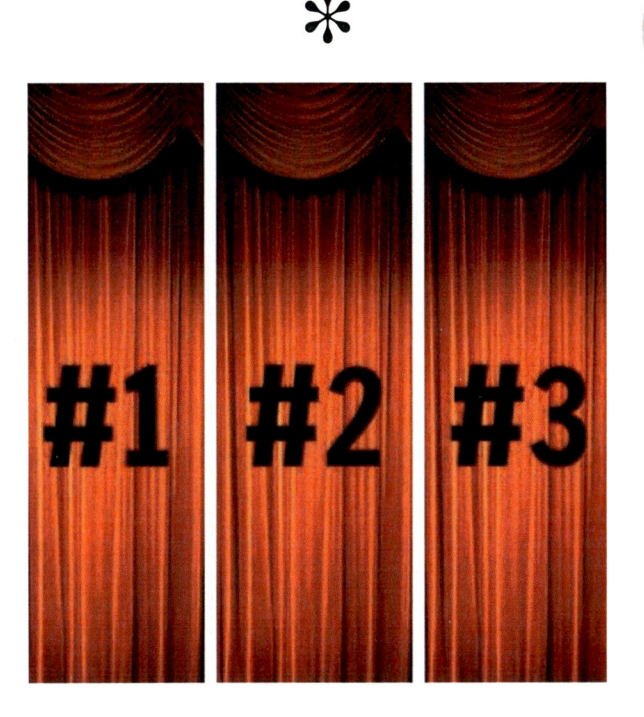

✻

On game shows there are never four curtains or doors. Only 3. Call it luck if you may, but the last door I had to open for pain relief was one more door, Door #4. I really, really hoped Door #4 was a grand prize and I would win the showcase showdown! I researched the procedure of the radiofrequency ablation a lot and spoke to others as well. Any and all information was beneficial for me. The radiofrequency ablation is considered a minor procedure. I never thought of it as minor- that was far from my thinking.

Radiofrequency Ablation is:

Cervical radiofrequency ablation involves using heat to burn the nerve tissue so the nerves cannot transmit pain signals to the brain.

The doctor will use X-rays (the fluoroscope, camera the technician will hold to guide the procedure and placement) to guide twin, insulated needles to the proper place next to the nerve. A tiny electrode is placed inside the needle. A small radiofrequency current is directed to the center of the branch nerve/the joint capsule for 60 to 90 seconds. The radiofrequency waves make heat. This destroys the nerve tissue that is sending the pain signals to the brain. Repeat the procedure at another level or area of the cervical spine. I had 3 levels performed.

The procedure is done with sterile technique to minimize the risk of infection.

After the procedure, you are taken to a recovery area. You aren't on a stretcher though. You get up and walk to the recovery room dawning the ugly gown. The nurses will monitor you and be sure you do not have an allergic reaction. You will be allowed to leave once you are stable.

You should rest for about 24 hours. And during this time not drive a car. I got to say, I never heard anyone say not to drive a car to or from this procedure.

This is what a pamphlet I read said about after the procedure: "You may feel more pain for several days after the procedure. Your doctor may give you additional pain-relieving medications until this goes away. There may be some swelling or bruising where the needle was inserted. A cold pack will help reduce the swelling". I got to say again, I remember this part I read, but never gave the level of pain much thought. I would have liked to seen big words to catch my attention. Like, overwhelming pain, bring you to your knees pain, stuff like that!

Cervical radiofrequency ablation is not permanent. With time, the nerves will regenerate, and the pain can sometimes return. Fingers crossed.

October 2019 and the day is here. I am nervous. I was only happy because the highways were dry, no snow. Away I go, distracting my nervousness with some Blue October music, only happy thoughts now.

I arrive on time and make my way through the check in and gown up. I will never get use to a gown. I am feeling gross and not just from this gown. I'm getting really nervous and feel the nerves all nestled in my stomach. When the doctor came into the room and sat down to explain the procedure answer questions it wasn't long before my blood pressure went down and I had confidence in myself I can do this. Let's open Door #4, Bob.

The technician brings me in the room to have me lie on table and get positioned. Deep breath in. And exhale. Physician walks in. I'm good still. This particular physician is known to be the best in city at this procedure so I'm trying to draw off that and the successful outcome of today's minor procedure.

First big needle of lidocaine comes in contact with my neck area. He does around 4 different spots to numb the area. Now the procedure begins. I'm focused like predator on its prey. I don't move. I don't talk. I don't curse. I focus. I lied. I did curse.

I knew each step he was doing. He kept talking to me at each of the steps. It helped. And I knew I was closer and closer to having it finished. I had a lot of lidocaine from start to finish so I was pretty frozen.

Forty-five minutes had passed when I heard these three words. You are done. Can I get a amen!!!! I did it!! I got up stepped down and walked to recovery area. I laid down for 10 minutes then got dressed and left. Nobody asked if I had a ride home, I should have. After 10 minutes of driving the pain hit me like a ton of bricks. I was in f*cken agony the rest of the way home. Amen my ass. "What in tarnation is this," I'm thinking to myself. I don't remember watching any videos like what I was experiencing. I get home and head to a bottle of pills. Tramadol was the prescription I had filled. I took as prescribed and felt some relief that was temporary then I took more when needed. The muscle pain was horrible. I was not expecting this. I had a 9/10 pain level. After 7 days of this pain, I went to our emergency department. The doctor that I saw was not up with this procedure so I told him what I had done. He said I had a lot of swelling, redness and moderate to severe pain associated with muscle soreness and muscle spasms. I was given some Tramacet for 7 days only that would provide some decrease in the swelling and decrease the intense pain. I took it for 7 days and noticed it did get somewhat better in the pain department, but not an instant relief. I figured I was in for the long haul with this and I was right.

It took a good three months for the procedure pain to stop and actually feel normal again which was only pre-ablation normal. I had work to do now in the physiotherapy department. I kept my spirits up while recovering, but looking back on it, I don't know how I did. I kick myself for not taking the rest time I needed. The results of this minor procedure were good. I was numb back of base of skull and along neck. That underlying nerve pain was gone. Now to get used to the numbness, which to me was a trade off, but worth it. Fast forward a couple of years now and the procedure was successful, but was not permanent. I am not seeking to have the procedure repeated at this point. I feel so much better right now, I just want to continue with physio and massage.

Just say no to drugs...

✼

I didn't have to say no to drugs...the pain killer kind. My family doctor did that for me. He never once prescribed any pain pills for me, other doctors did for post procedure pain, but my family doctor who I have seen for over 35 years never showed me his prescription pad. Although initially, he did prescribe something to help me sleep, Trazadone, which had some pain-relieving properties. It did help with getting to sleep, but not the pain. After several months on this sleep medication, the affect was somewhat wearing off or the pain was too much all the time and it over rode it's effects to help me sleep.

I didn't know really know why and really didn't want a giant dosage to bring me down. That sounded like an animal ranger darting a rhino, no thanks! After about a year, I stopped taking the medication and tried other things to help with sleep. I started back on melatonin which was helpful prior to this injury, but I didn't get the same effect now. I had troubles falling asleep, staying asleep and getting a restful sleep. I started to read about meditation for the insomnia and thought I would try this route. Muscle relaxation meditation involves paying attention to your body, tensing and relaxing each muscle one by one, from head to toe. Accompanied with some soothing music and a pink light in the room, at times I could allow all the muscles to shoosh while I tried to fall asleep. There are other techniques in meditation, but I never tried those, maybe I should or could have, but I didn't feel the need to go deeper into the meditation world. I also tried tapping for quite some time which is used to disrupt the unbalanced energy your body has. I quite liked tapping. I would also just stay up late in hopes exhaustion would allow some deep sleep for a few hours. I did try the float tank or Sensory Deprivation Therapy. They say or suggest that spending time floating in a sensory deprivation tank may have some benefits in healthy people, such as muscle relaxation, better sleep, decrease in pain, and decreased stress and anxiety. My shoulders hurt so bad and it only kept me in a tighter state of tension. It wasn't for me; maybe later on it will have some benefits.

For some relief in the muscle relaxant department, I was prescribed some little pills, yellow, look like houses... Ah, I remember those little devils! It was the muscle relaxant prescription, Flexeril. They sound like what I need, but will they do the trick? The answer to that is a big fat NO. I took one or two muscle relaxant (in the afternoon) and was out like a light for hours and hours. Apparently, I had supper in between the sleeping and out of it feeling. I tried to take them just before going to sleep, but no effect on me. I don't think I took anymore after that and finally just chucked them in the garbage, they just weren't for me. When my muscles were relaxed and I did get some restful sleep, I was super happy, this usually occurred two days a week. The other five days of the week I was just bloody miserable. I craved a good night sleep.

The only consistent and available medication I have taken for the pain is a wack of Advil. The liquid blue gels, or liquid gold as I liked to call them. It reduced the pain. It never cut the pain off. And no prescription was required. I was, and am, well aware of the many cons to pain killers, but damn...there were so many days that were unbearable. I also tried over the counter creams and patches, but none worked until a nurse I worked with told me about a cream that I could purchase and it was an over-the-counter medicated cream that would numb the pain in the affected area. The name of it was Maxilene and it helped a lot. I saved it for the grouchy muscle pain days. It was enough to take the edge off.

Now, when I had the radio frequency ablation procedure, this was a whole different level of pain that came my way. If I knew the pain level and recovery from that procedure was going to be such a long and painful time, I still would have done it. The medication I was prescribed for this procedure was Tramadol and was a very effective medication for pain. It cut the pain off and in my brain, I had no pain. I was given the Tramadol with some refills and I used those refills too. I never abused the pills. I had leftover because I didn't need the full dosage amount prescribed as time went on. I saved these little nuggets of gold for bad days which I was sure were still to come.

I was told at my first neurologist/Botox appointment that I should never have been given the Tramadol as I could have become addicted. When I took this medication, it cut the pain off and I didn't get a high effect, but was simply "very happy" the pain stopped. Is that high? I don't think the happiness I felt was like being high, the drug kind of high. It was my happy high. I never took enough at once to get the effect. After this many years I can say I am glad I didn't have pain killers at my beck and call. But I sure did love them when I had to take and the affect they had on my pain. I still have 4 tablets left and have not used any in many months. That's how precious they are to me. Emergency use only, like for the Indiana Jones ride at Disneyland. I guess my family doctor did the right thing by never giving me pain killers. Side note, I did also have a go with pot wafers and gummies, but no real pain reducing effect came from taking this. I find the fact the legalization of cannabis in Canada now dampens my want to use after being illegal in the country for many decades.

Analyze this... psychology...how does that make you feel?

✱

As funny as we have made the saying, "and how does that make you feel," it's a valid question to begin your journey with getting a healthy mind back and navigating the road to it.

I had started to think that my frustration and irritability was getting the best of me dealing with this pain and having some emotional baggage as well. My emotions were all over the place. I wasn't handling the pain well and really didn't know what way to go at this point, it's been over a year of mostly pain and frustration. When I was feeling okay, my mood was somewhat normal, emphasis on the somewhat. After any successful physio appointment, I remember feeling more able to attack the work I needed to do with this injury which was doing the physiotherapy exercises and being consistent with them. But the good feeling didn't last long enough and I felt defeated again and again. Same shitty cycle over and over with this pain which seems to be fitting into a chronic condition. I was not ready to settle into this cycle.

I decided to go talk with someone in the fall of 2018. I was referred to someone close to my town which was fantastic, no driving to the city. My first appointment went well. I felt very comfortable talking to this lady. The office was warm and inviting as was Miss Judy. I wasn't sure where or how I was going to start I just really wanted to vomit all my feelings out. This wasn't just about the pain anymore. I had feelings of frustration, anger, boredom, sadness, helplessness and frustration, or did I say that last one already? There was also one other emotion, its' name was guilt.

Part of my guilty feelings were tied to the days I missed work mixed with some people who I felt had doubt in this injury. Even though I missed very little work. (Because I always made the missed work up in the evening or weekends) I would always feel guilty when I did call in sick. Calling in sick in the workplace is just plain uncomfortable anyways. I always felt they didn't believe me unless I had laryngitis or a really bad cold, you know, something that was palpable over the phone. So when I called in sick because the pain was so horrible on this day and I didn't know what caused the flare up, the guilt kicked in.

I always felt some just didn't understand or want to believe the cycle of this pain. And a lot of people who don't have any experience with chronic pain tend to not open their mind to the person who has it. Those people tend to leave some remark that in turn leaves you thinking less of yourself and you start to question everything and try harder to prove your injury. Believe me, when someone says, "Well, you look good" that is not what I was looking for. Of course, I want to look good, but I want to feel the same, and I rarely did, FEEL good. It took extra time in my days to get up and get ready and look okay. I would also start to just lie when someone said, "how are you?" I would automatically say, "good." There's your answer, now go away, try not to come back either with that same question.

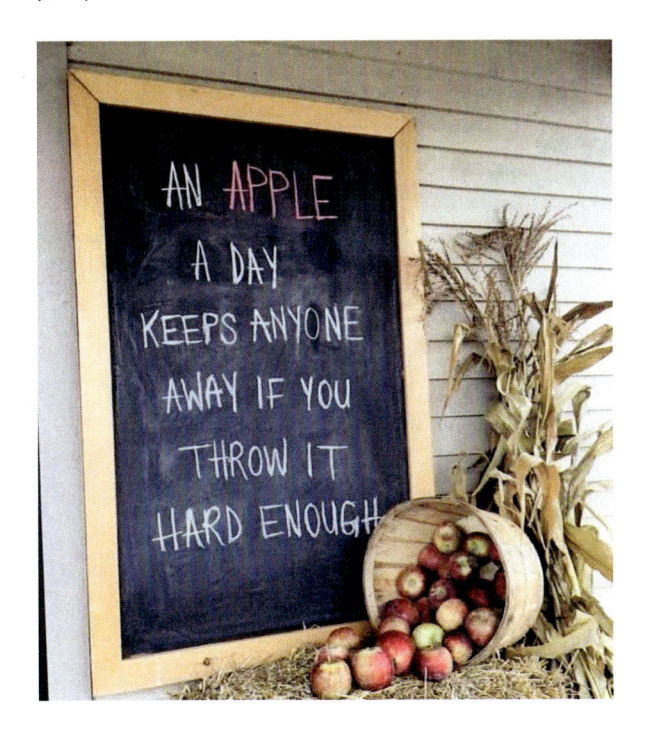

I had to listen to some coworkers tell me, "there's nothing wrong with you. It's in your head. Go try walking more." Even when some people never or some just stopped asking how I was over time, it messed with my head. I became a person trying to justify this injury. I felt like I had my hand in the cookie jar all the damn time. It was exhausting. This fed me more of my anger, frustration and disappointment. Talking to Miss Judy was the place I could let her know anything I was feeling. Our sessions touched on all aspects of things I was somewhat struggling with. I was juggling appointments galore, too much driving, working full-time, life in general, while this pain followed me like a stray puppy. Omg, if I let this pain follow me, I would have a boarding kennel full of dogs. Not a bad thing, the dogs, but Miss Judy was about finding solutions in all these areas.

We focused on pain relief and what I could do on my own. Like getting the cup of tea out of a microwave. The microwave stopped when the cup was in the back, well that hurt grabbing all the way in! We found a solution and that was to stop microwave when my cup was in the front! Silly sounding, but at this point, I knew all the breaks I gave my pain would benefit me and my anger/frustration.

These types of conversations showed me the kindness and genuine thoughtfulness Miss Judy gave our sessions. I was also given tools in the form of readings, like surveys, measures and questionnaires which I fully embraced and did. I learned a lot in all of our sessions and learned more about myself than I really knew.

My focus wasn't what it should have been. Pain tends to lay a blanket of haze over your focus. It took me many sessions to understand and believe in myself and my feelings. Shit it took me many sessions to remember what she was discussing with me the last session. These sessions and talks were getting me to the place to not only voice feelings, but first believe this chronic pain I had to deal with was real. My feelings counted and I had the right to express and follow through on what I expressed. I couldn't figure out why I found it hard to do. I have always said how I felt throughout my life, and yes, sometimes unfiltered. Seriously who hasn't become somewhat unhinged at something in their life and left the 'unfilter' volume up?

I also knew in certain situations to not say what was really on my mind because of the negative effects it could have. I came to the realization that a situation I never imagined would come my way or I was trying to maybe ignore or think it would get better, was here. I kept to myself and became quiet. This is how I was feeling now. To be quiet. If I chose to say how I felt, I would be seen in a negative light. I felt it best to keep quiet and carry on. I was carrying all this baggage and it was weighing me down little by little.

And speaking of baggage, I use to pull a cart that carried binders and equipment when I use to go to clinic at work and see patients for assessments. As time went on pulling this cart, I would have to leave earlier and earlier from my office to do the walk to the clinic. I would need to stop once or twice on the way due to pain.

On the way back, I had to stop three or four times and just sit and be still. After months of this I asked two co-workers (great assistants in my job) for a big favor. The favor was to pull that bloody cart over for me; I just couldn't do it anymore. One said, "absolutely" (I predicated that answer), the other didn't want to at all (I didn't predict that answer and the extra dialogue that came with it). And because I never really wanted to ask that of them and have any disappointment, I didn't give a crap about the negative answer. This was the moment when I realized, little by little, I had been adding more me to my confidence jar, thanks to Miss Judy, and all the insight and guidance on in our sessions she had been giving me. This was big. I gave myself my permission now. I gave myself permission to take me back and do what was right, do what made sense now. The first obstacle I faced was driving to an office job that immediately sent my body into a state of pain; therefore, I can't be driving to the city 45 minutes each way. The job role was not going to allow me to work from home and I was also not going to further engage in a power struggle at my job. I'm too old for that shit. The decision I needed to make was not easy. I loved my job and was good at it. When I did make the decision to leave, I wrote a small list of things I needed to do. I also wrote out the perfect job for Whiplash Shelley. My decision to leave did not disappoint. I found a job in the same field and I work from home now. No more long daily drives and no more guilt. How refreshing and revitalizing!! This wasn't a band-aid fix, it was a permanent fix.

> A HA Moment
>
> Know when to hold 'em
> Know when to fold em
>
> When the volley becomes too toxic
> It's time to walk off the court
>
> There is no reward for settling for something you don't want

Miss Judy was proud of me and this accomplishment, and I was proud of me! I am finding difficult situations easy to make right for myself.

Psychology encounters are healthy goals to understand our cognitive, emotional and behaviour processes that we face in our daily lives. I always look forward to my appointments. Indeed, always time well spent.

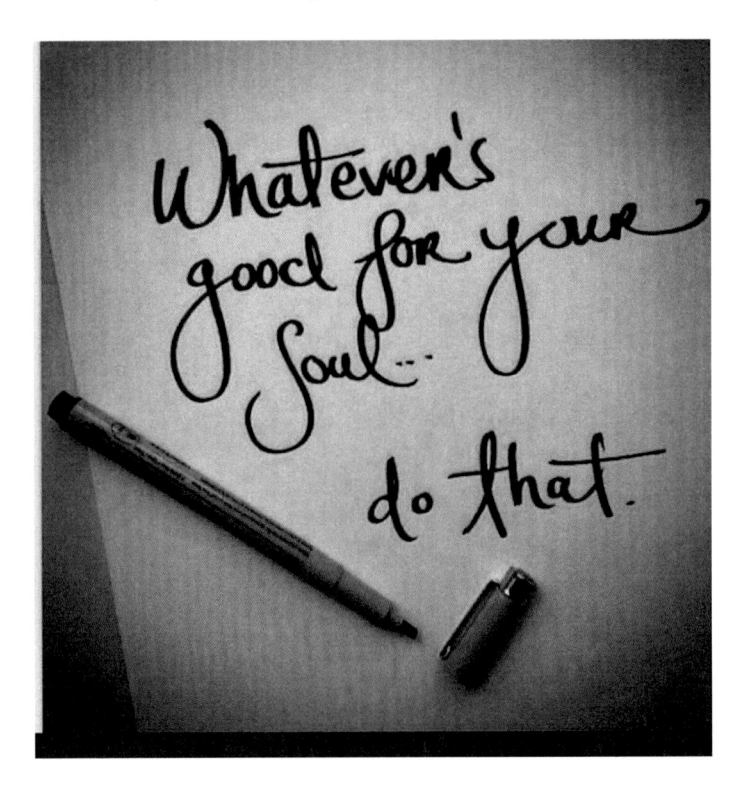

We've booked you an IME Bitch...

*

The IME is: Independent Medical Examination.

The insurance company will arrange and pay for this medical examination. The insurance company typically selects an assessor who has historically provided them with conclusions that benefit them, not you. These assessors are physicians. In my opinion, these physicians are in bed with the insurance companies.

My option was to not go and be cut off the insurance claim or go and be cut off the insurance claim if the physician found my injury to not require further treatment. Up until this point my insurance claim was only covering the cost of physiotherapy and the dental portion for my jaw injury (TMJD). There was nothing extra coming from them. I also knew from early on there would be no friendly conversations with this big insurance company.

Because I had nothing to hide and was not faking this, of course I set up the appointment. The insurance company was very surprised I called and booked it. I don't know if that comment was a part of their theatrics/game or they were just being stupid. The appointment was set up and it was to take place in the city at a physiotherapy business.

I was not nervous for the appointment.

I arrived on time and sat in the waiting room ready to get this over with. I was put into a regular exam room and waited for the doctor. A few minutes later the doctor enters with a pretend smile. Her pretend smile was not the only thing she pretended. She pretended to care as she interviewed me. For the history portion of the appointment, I was quite relaxed giving her answers as she asked and never stalled or had to think about any of the answers. All of the answers were given truthfully by me. Half way through this history portion of the IME I kind of was thinking she might have some "care" in her with the wee bit of empathy she showed. She actually gave me a Kleenex at one point as it was getting emotional when I spoke to the things, I wasn't able to "just" do anymore and how much pain I was having and the likes of dealing with it. In hindsight, I should have stuffed the Kleenex in her mouth so I didn't have to listen to anymore of her bullshit.

I was surprised I showed that side of me in front of her. But I thought she was sympathizing with me and how the emotional sides of pain affected me. I was wrong. The review/interview of the accident and treatments thus far really didn't take that long, I would say 15 or so minutes. The paperwork/questions were geared toward a negative outcome anyhow. The questions they asked, whether you answered yes or no, always gave the insurance company a way out. After her history portion we went on to the examination portion. This part was joke but not a funny joke. I was fully clothed from head to toe. Even kept my sneakers on! I didn't see any gowns and thought she was going to leave and get one, but she didn't. Fine by me. She got me to bend and stretch a bit. I emphasize a bit because the whole exam was about 5 minutes. Twice she had contact with my body. First was to run the Wartenburg Pinwheel over my foot with my shoes on.

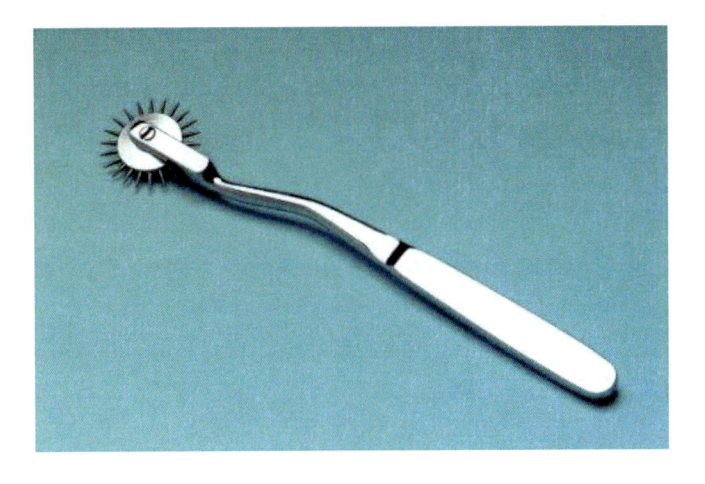

I felt nothing. Not sure what she would be remarking on with that test. Patient can't feel her toes? Doctor can't see the patient's toes? Second contact was when she "booped" her finger on the back of my head as I faced the wall. This is a dictionary meaning of the word boop: A gentle or playful tap or strike. Her index finger had the least amount of pressure, but it was enough and on the right spot to cause me to react as she had booped on a tender spot. And that's all that was done. I wanted to ask her to feel my shoulders, feel my jaw, and feel my freakin' head. Feel where it hurts! I have one word for her examination, unethical. I left and went to my car and knew I had a big F for a mark. I started with an F though so it didn't matter. Just like going or not going, their mind is made up before you go.

Within a few weeks, the IME report was in the hands of my insurance company. The insurance claim agent called the physiotherapy place first and told them I would no longer be covered for further treatment. Two days later they called me and said I would no longer be receiving further treatment from this accident claim. This decision smelled, the same smell when you drive by a pig farm. Car insurance is a big business and fighting their decision was a mountain I didn't want to climb. But reporting the unethical doctor for a shawdy exam was. I told my family doctor about the decision from insurance and he suggested and supported I write a letter to the college of physicians and surgeons. I have not done it though. I feel too much time has passed now to send my thoughts to the college of physicians/surgeons and like my dad always said, "what goes around, comes around." I believe hers will come around.

Fast forward a week and I receive the official letter from insurance company explaining I'm cut off blah, blah and pretty much don't call us again. Are you wondering if I canceled my car insurance? Not only did I cancel car, but the house insurance as well. Well over 20-year clients to this insurance company now only to part with irreconcilable differences. I dedicated a chapter in this book with some fine artwork to really capture the flavor and smells of this insurance company.

It was disheartening to know insurance didn't have my back nor did the doctor. I'm the one left with the pain, continuing treatment and trying to navigate the health system in our province that imposes too many road blocks as it is.

Botox...not just for celebrities

*

My family doctor referred me to a neurologist in March 2020. The referral appointment didn't take long to get at all which I was surprised at because getting a specialist appointment usually has a few months waitlist. When I received the doctors name, I googled him to check reviews. The reviews weren't normal, some reviews were good, but lots were not good. Initially, my 'spidy' senses said, "don't go." A few weeks before my appointment with the neurologist, I called the physiatrist to ask some questions about Botox in general. He said I would be a good candidate, but also said that Botox weakened the muscles. He then asked who the neurologist was to which I answered. He immediately said, "just don't read the reviews." Too late, I already had.

To keep everyone happy, or not be difficult I think, I kept the appointment with this neurologist. In April of 2020 I went to see him. I didn't go in thinking anything at all, I would see for myself, no pre-judgement. Well, shit. Just, for shit's sake. First thing you notice is an assistant that accompanies him to all his appointments with female patients. I knew within 10 seconds there was more to the not good reviews and as I would read later, there indeed was. This appointment made me uncomfortable, but I continued with it. The neurologist stated that I have migraines and would benefit from Botox. The end result of this initial consult would be to start Botox injections for migraines and to reduce the tight muscles in the shoulders. I agreed to this, mainly for the tight muscles. I didn't agree I suffered from migraines though. To this day, I do not think I had migraines, just frequent headaches which always made sense to me.

Prior to getting to my first Botox appointment I had to stop at the pharmacy and get the boxes of Botox as well as the needles/syringes. I was still thinking, I could change my mind right now and not go to this neurologist appointment. But I picked up the filled prescription and drove to the city. During my drive I was still unsure if I should attend. I could change my mind and do a U-turn right now! "I could find another doctor," I thought. I arrived on time and give them the Botox and now my nerves are taking over and I really just wanted to turn around and walk out. I get called into the exam room where I see a metal tray and they have filled 4 or 5 syringes with some Botox. I was instructed to sit up on exam table. No gown and I would have flat out refused with this doctor. Then the doctor just starts the procedure, NO warning. The injections into back of my head in 5 or 6 different spots went so fast, f-bombs exploded out of my mouth quick, loud and with intention. The injections hurt in the shoulders, but the ones in the face were not as bad. It was five long minutes of injections that hurt like hell! I left with instructions which were to sit up a minimum of 4 hours. By the time I got home all I wanted to do was lay down. I took some Advil for the pain and watched the clock until I could lie down. I didn't feel well overall, nausea and just blah. The rest of the day and next day I felt the same, blah. I felt I had a nagging small headache waiting for permission to explode into a bad headache.

In the months from first injection to second one coming up, I noticed nothing different in headache amounts or relaxing of tight muscles. Felt the same really, but I don't think the first session would have shown any vast improvement. Next appointment is here, it's three months later. Performed the same routine getting the Botox, driving with dread to the appointment that morning. But this appointment was odd. When I arrived, the waiting room was empty. I was not greeted by receptionist at beginning or saw any of them at the end of this appointment. The neurologist came out of their office and called me in. I sit down and know that something is not normal right away. The doctor was overly professional, so much, it was too weird. I see their assistant with the metal tray and she has already started to load the weapons with Botox. The session was unremarkable, meaning no change for the positions of all the needles, nor the intensity of pain they inflicted. As I was getting up and putting my shoes on, the neurologist said to me that they wished me well and goodbye. Can't scratch my head because of pain, but HUH? What does that mean? For sure, something is going on. I left, knowing I wouldn't be coming back, I'll find someone else.

It would be a couple weeks later when I get a call from a doctor at my place of work that proceeds to tell me this neurologist has had their medical practice suspended. I wanted to vomit. The College of Physician & Surgeons was doing an investigation. I thanked the physician for this information and very nicely said I would not be going back even if they are reinstated to practice again.

I went and saw my family doctor for another neurology referral. We didn't really talk about the incident, but I did open with WTH and those were my only words on it.

I was referred again and went to the second neurologist appointment, but I did not get to see the neurologist. Instead, I saw a general practitioner. Nothing wrong with this, but I wasn't sure why no neurologist. This general practitioner sounded like she was well versed in the Botox protocol for headaches and muscle spasms/tightness. I'm on board with this then, let's continue the Botox. First appointment went off without a hitch; I prepared myself for the pain. After a full year of doing these Botox injections, I decided on my own I didn't want to continue anymore. I did have positive results in my shoulders and liked that, but I was feeling weaker/fatigue in my shoulders all the time and I didn't want that.

I Cancelled My Car Insurance Policy... and House Insurance Policy

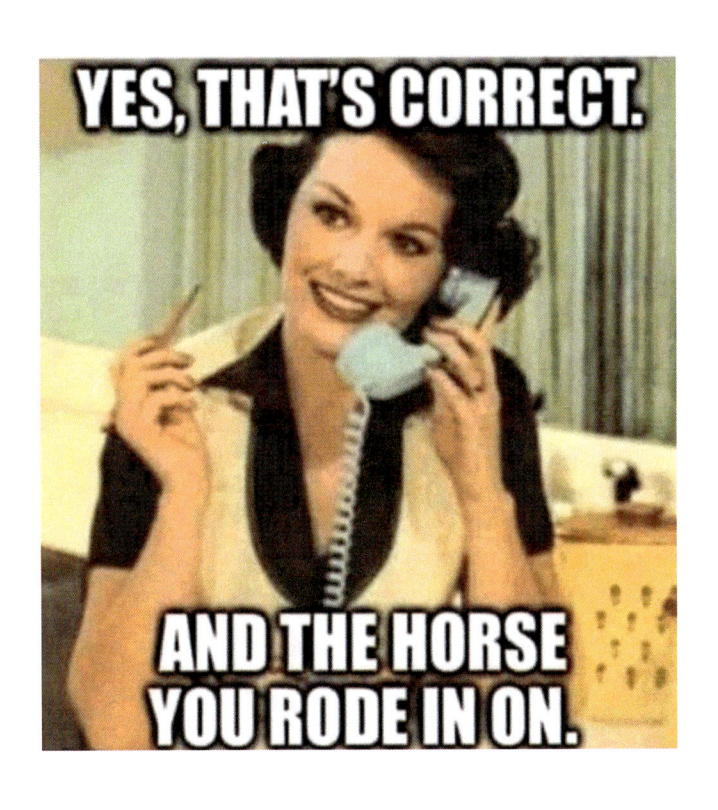

YES, THAT'S CORRECT.

AND THE HORSE YOU RODE IN ON.

Friend...such a simple word for one of the great necessities of life

✶

Always have time to listen. Always give good advice. These are my closet friends.

Our friendships are 40 to 50 years old. "This stupid injury is really testing our friendship," is what I believed. I often thought that I am talking too much about my pain, being too negative, but, it was hard to control that at times. We are all still friends and I feel closer to them now than ever before.

They always knew what to say to ease or bring me off the ledge so to speak.

I would text to say can't talk too sore in mouth or say don't make me laugh if we talk. That would never happen, ever. Our shits and giggles always go too far, and we like it that way. They had their own ways to help me cope. Coping is really turning shit into sunshine! Weather forecast, divine.

We visit when we can. We talk all the time. We travel together. Good friends, all blessed.

I've been told that if any of us were to go into an elderly care facility together our kids may be getting phone calls.

Phone calls because we are getting out of hand and they may need to re-home us if we don't settle down! I can hardly wait for that time to come!

Truthfully, I couldn't imagine going through some of the shitty dark days without them. And I couldn't imagine going through all the sunshine days without them!

Finish Line:

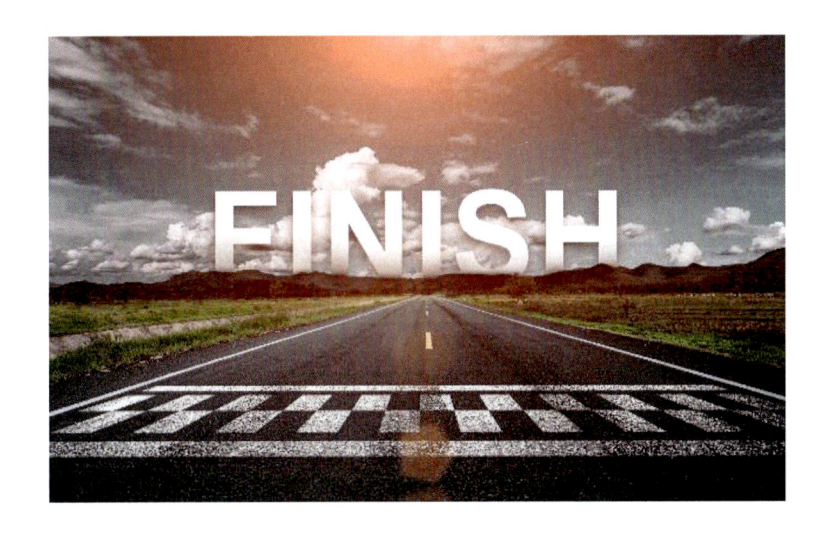

✲

It's been quite a trip. Lots of different roads to travel to get to this part. The finish for me is being out of active treatments I had to investigate to mitigate this chronic pain. Maybe I didn't have the traditional finish line cross for first, second or third place, but my staggered victory of pain relief was having them crossover into other victories.

I am having more happy life moments now and that is a huge gauge of where my pain level is at this point.

I am most certainly a big advocate of physiotherapy and needles! Bring 'em on, they work! I will be a client of physiotherapy for a while longer and even after, tune ups will be required.

I am a grandmother now. I'll be doing lots more with him now, he's already Mickey Mouse obsessed so no training required. I remember that I could hardly pack this guy around when he was little.

I am an author now, good or bad, an excellent therapeutic journey for myself.

I am never going to look back and regret this pathway, highway, by-way or any of the ways I chose or was guided to take or try.

To order more copies of this book, find books by other Canadian authors, or make inquiries about publishing your own book, contact PageMaster at:

PageMaster Publication Services Inc.
11340-120 Street, Edmonton, AB T5G 0W5
books@pagemaster.ca
780-425-9303

catalogue and e-commerce store
PageMasterPublishing.ca/Shop